The Complete Erectile Dysfunction Handbook

Advanced Guide to Fixing Weak Erections and Boosting Male Sexual Health to Overcome ED, Enhance Low Libido, and Improve Your Sexual Confidence Forever

Erickson Tom Brown

Copyright

Copyright © 2024 Erickson Tom Brown.

Table of Contents

Introduction

mpotence has become a significant issue that impacts not just physical health but also self-esteem and mental well-being. Many people suffer in silence because of the shame associated with this problem, believing they fall short of what society expects of them. Male traits like strength, virility, and confidence are frequently associated with masculinity in society. Men may struggle with feelings of guilt and inadequacy when these qualities deteriorate, which can worsen the issue by creating a vicious cycle of anxiety. It is essential to understand that impotence is an emotional struggle that calls for vulnerability and bravery; it is not merely a medical ailment. By offering methods for overcoming impotence and boosting self-esteem, this book seeks to empower men.

Description

We can start eliminating the stigma and reinterpreting what it means to be an empowered man by encouraging candid discussion and providing workable answers. We'll work together to examine the complexities of the mind-body link, the influence of lifestyle decisions, and the significance of emotional intelligence in re-establishing one's sense of self. As you set out on this path, remember that the first step to empowerment is admitting your difficulties. Let's examine these issues and discover the resources required to restore your well-being and self-assurance.

Chapter One

What Impotence Is All About

Millions of men worldwide have impotence, often known as erectile dysfunction (ED), which is still one of the most stigmatized and little-understood conditions in society. A deeper examination of impotence's multifaceted nature—including psychological and physical components—is necessary to comprehend it. The Aspects of the Body and the Mind Hormonal imbalances, long-term conditions like diabetes or heart disease, and adverse drug reactions are only a few of the physiological causes of impotence. These medical conditions might interfere with the body's normal functions, making it challenging to get or keep an erection. Effective remedies, from medical interventions to lifestyle modifications, can result from speaking with a healthcare professional.

Psychological and emotional aspects significantly influence sexual health. Stress, anxiety, and depression can all contribute to a vicious cycle in which the dread of impotence makes the illness worse. Particularly prevalent is performance anxiety, which causes problems in the present due to worries about performing poorly. Relational dynamics, self-perception, and prior experiences further weave this complex web of difficulties.

It also emphasises how crucial it is to treat the body and the intellect to find answers. Men can handle their condition more holistically if they acknowledge that impotence can result from a combination of psychological and physical issues.

Eliminating the Stigma

Many men feel alone and ashamed as a result of the stigma associated with impotence, which frequently inhibits candid conversation. The idea that sexual performance is a sign of masculinity has long been reinforced by society, which makes people feel inadequate when they experience erectile dysfunction. In addition to making mental suffering worse, this societal narrative deters males from getting treatment.

Destroying this stigma requires normalising discussions about impotence. Sexual health should be treated with the same degree of understanding and support as physical health issues, which are openly discussed and treated. Men who share their experiences can understand that impotence is a widespread problem rather than a particular shortcoming and find support in their battles. Creating a culture that embraces vulnerability is the first step in promoting openness. This entails being open and honest with friends and lovers, getting professional assistance when necessary, and realising that mental health is a crucial component of total well-being.

Redefining the story is essential as we set out on this quest to overcome impotence. Dealing with impotence is a show of courage and strength, not a sign of weakness. By working together, we can dispel the stigma and foster a more encouraging atmosphere where men are encouraged to ask for assistance and welcome their paths to better health and self-assurance. In the upcoming chapters, we shall examine doable methods for conquering impotence, emphasising lifestyle modifications, emotional intelligence, and forming dependable connections.

Understanding is the first step to empowerment, and you've already taken it.

Chapter 2

How Our Mind and Body Connection Affects Our Erection

One essential component of the human experience is the complex interaction between the mind and body, particularly when it comes to sexual performance. Addressing impotence requires an understanding of this relationship because mental and physical health are strongly correlated. The Impact of Mental Health on Sexual Performance Stress and anxiety frequently combine to form a complicated web that traps a man's confidence and fosters self-doubt. A performance that feels forced and strained can result from the persistent feelings of inadequacy taking precedence over desire during intimate moments. Fear of falling short of expectations may turn what should be a happy event into a battleground of anxiety, where the brain's constant chatter overpowers the body's natural reactions. Social conventions that associate masculinity with sexual aptitude frequently serve as fuel for this inner monologue. Men may become mired in a cycle of disappointment if they internalise these ideas.

A single erectile dysfunction incident can trigger widespread anxiety, which feeds back into the idea that one is inadequate. One's capacity to participate entirely in intimate times might be seriously hampered by this skewed self-perception, which can increase feelings of loneliness and annoyance.

Furthermore, stress can negatively impact sexual function, whether it comes from relationships, the workplace, or life's obstacles. Sexual arousal is one of the non-essential processes that are deprived of energy due to the body's stress reaction. Prolonged stress can exacerbate impotence by causing hormonal imbalances, exhaustion, and a decreased libido. In addition to being advantageous, mental health treatment is essential for re-establishing a healthy sexual life.

Techniques for Meditation and Mindfulness

Mindfulness and meditation provide effective methods to break this cycle of anxiety and develop a healthier relationship with oneself. By encouraging people to centre themselves in the here and now, mindfulness helps people release their anxious thoughts. Concentrating on breathing and bodily sensations can establish a calm mental environment where anxieties dissolve, creating space for closeness and connection. Breathing techniques like mindful breathing entail taking a deep breath, holding it for a short while and then slowly releasing it.

This small gesture might help a person become more grounded in the here and now by calming the mind and enabling one to concentrate on bodily sensations rather than performance pressures. Even spending a short period of time each day on this activity can greatly increase one's sense of confidence and serenity. Additionally, meditation is a mental haven. It provides a haven from the bustle of everyday life, allowing people to develop inner clarity and serenity.

Men who regularly meditate can become more aware of their thoughts and feelings, which will enable them to face difficulties with composure and resilience, whether they relate to relationships or their self-image. Methods such as guided imagery can be instrumental.

Imagine a tranquil setting, like a calm forest or a beach. By using all of the senses, this visualization can strengthen feelings of calm and serve as a potent diversion from unpleasant thoughts.

A feeling of acceptance and connection can also be fostered by practicing loving-kindness meditation, which entails thinking pleasant thoughts to oneself and others. Over time, incorporating these techniques into everyday routines might result in significant changes.

Studies have demonstrated that practising mindfulness and meditation can improve emotional regulation, lessen the symptoms of anxiety and depression, and improve general well-being. Men can better handle the demands of intimacy as they grow more aware of their thoughts and emotions.

As we review the following chapters, remember that taking care of your mental health is essential to conquering impotence and regaining your confidence, not just a side endeavour. The path to empowerment starts on the inside, where self-love and mindfulness can grow and create a healthy environment for mental and physical health. You can improve your sexual experiences, develop a more positive self-image, and eventually change the way you and your partner interact by adopting these behaviours.

Chapter 3

Foods and Exercises That Improve Sexual Health

Changes in lifestyle are essential for overcoming impotence and boosting confidence. Men can develop a healthy body and mind by emphasising stress management, sleep, fitness, and nutrition. This will pave the way for better sexual health and general well-being. Exercise and Nutrition: Activities and Foods That Promote Sexual Health and Self-Esteem The Basis of Sexual Health: Nutrition Sexual function is one of the many bodily functions significantly impacted by the foods we eat. Blood flow, hormone levels, and general energy levels can all be improved with a nutritious, well-balanced diet—all of which are critical for getting and keeping an erection.

1. Fruits

Vitamins, minerals, and antioxidants in fruits and vegetables promote cardiovascular health. Kale, spinach, citrus fruits, and berries are particularly healthy. Citrulline, for example, is found in watermelon and may help increase blood flow.

2. Good Fats:
Omega-3 fatty acids, which are present in walnuts, flaxseeds, and fish (such as salmon and mackerel), support a healthy circulatory system. Erectile function depends on heart health, which is supported by these lipids.

3. Whole Grains:
Quinoa, brown rice, and oats are nutritious foods that help keep blood sugar levels steady. Hormonal balance and general energy levels depend on these.

4. Lean protein:
Beans, lentils, turkey, and chicken promote hormone production and muscle health. Protein is essential for healing and general endurance.

5. Nuts and Seeds:
Zinc and vitamin E, found in almonds, pistachios, and pumpkin seeds, are

associated with higher testosterone levels and better sexual health.

6. **Dark Chocolate**:

Dark chocolate, packed with antioxidants, benefits sexual function by lowering blood pressure and increasing blood flow. A Mediterranean diet, which emphasizes fruits, vegetables, whole grains, seafood, and healthy fats, has improved erectile function and general health.

Foods and exercises that boost sexual health

Regular exercise is another essential component of a healthy lifestyle. In addition to improving physical health, it also improves body image and self-esteem, two important aspects of sexual confidence.

1. Cardiovascular Exercise:

Exercises that increase heart health and blood circulation include jogging, cycling, swimming, and brisk walking. To get and keep an erection, you need a robust cardiovascular system.

2. Strength Training:

Lifting weights or performing bodyweight workouts can increase testosterone levels and build muscle mass. Exercises that improve general strength and vigour include push-ups, deadlifts, and squats.

3. Kegel exercises:
Although they are frequently linked to women, men might benefit from them. By strengthening the pelvic floor muscles, these workouts help improve erectile function and ejaculation control. Determine which muscles are used to stop urinating, contract them for a short while, and then relax to conduct Kegel exercises. Every day, try to complete three sets of ten to fifteen reps.

4. Yoga Exercise:
Yoga and stretching can help people de-stress and relax. Some yoga postures, such as the Bridge pose and the Cobra stance, can increase sexual function by increasing blood flow to the pelvic region.

5. Mind-Body Exercises:
Practices like Pilates and tai chi emphasise body and breath awareness, lowering anxiety and enhancing mental clarity while promoting sexual health. Incorporating regular exercise into your schedule doesn't have to be complicated. Try to get at least 150 minutes of moderate aerobic exercise and two strength training sessions every

week. Maintaining a schedule when engaging in fun activities is more straightforward, which improves mental and physical health.

The Importance of Rest

The Influence of Sleep The importance of sleep for general wellness and sexual health is sometimes overlooked. Hormonal balance, mood stability, and cognitive function depend on getting enough sleep. Reduced libido, elevated tension, and anxiety are all consequences of sleep deprivation that can exacerbate impotence.

Sleep Management

1. Create a Sleep Routine:
Your body's internal clock is regulated when you go to bed and wake up simultaneously every day, making falling and remaining asleep more straightforward.

2. Establish a Calm Environment:
Keep your bedroom calm, cold, and dark to create a haven for restful sleep. Consider using white noise machines, earplugs, or blackout curtains if necessary.

3. Reduce Screen Time Before Bed:

Computers, tablets, and phones emit blue light, disrupting melatonin generation. To encourage healthier sleep, try to switch off devices at least an hour before bed.

4. Mindful Wind-Down Rituals:
Include soothing exercises like reading, light stretching, or a warm bath in your bedtime routine. Additionally, mindfulness exercises can help calm the mind and prepare the body for a good night's sleep.

5. Limit Stimulants:
Limit your nicotine and caffeine intake, particularly in the hours before bed. These drugs might cause restlessness and interfere with sleep cycles.

6. Seek Professional Assistance:
If your sleep problems continue, you might want to speak with a healthcare professional. Sexual function and overall health can be significantly impacted by sleep disorders like sleep apnea.

6 Ways to Reduce Stress to Achieve Better Erection

Striking a Balance Stress is an unavoidable part of our fast-paced, modern lives. However, long-term stress can negatively impact physical and mental health, including sexual function. Regaining confidence and self-empowerment requires effective stress management.

The following are practical methods for managing stress:
1. Frequent Exercise:
As was already said, exercise is an effective way to reduce stress. It lowers anxiety levels and releases endorphins, the body's natural mood enhancers.

2. Meditation & Mindfulness:
Including mindfulness practices into your everyday routine can facilitate a sense of peace. Techniques like gradual muscle relaxation, deep breathing, and meditation can also considerably decrease stress and anxiety.

3. Time management:
Prioritising and organising work can help reduce feelings of overwhelm. Use tools like planners or to-do lists to divide more complex undertakings into smaller, more doable chores.

4. Social Networks:
Having a network of encouraging friends and relatives might help you cope with stress. Sharing your ideas and feelings with

someone you can trust can facilitate connecting and receiving emotional support.

5. Interests and Hobbies:
Participating in enjoyable activities can offer a much-needed reprieve from the stresses of everyday life. Painting, gardening, or playing an instrument are examples of creative pursuits that might improve general well-being.

6. Professional Support:
If stress becomes intolerable, consulting a therapist or counsellor can offer helpful coping mechanisms and emotional support. In conclusion, resolving impotence and boosting confidence require adopting lifestyle modifications centred on stress management, sleep, fitness, and diet.

Men can build a strong foundation for sexual health and general empowerment by feeding their bodies healthful meals, exercising frequently, getting enough sleep, and handling stress well. Making deliberate decisions that respect the body and the mind is the first step towards regaining vitality. Making these adjustments will not only enhance your sexual health but also help you feel more confident and valuable in other facets of your life.

Chapter 4

Developing Emotional Intelligence

The key element of relational and personal well-being is emotional intelligence (EI), which significantly improves confidence and tackles problems like impotence. It includes the capacity for efficient understanding, control, and expression of emotions, all essential for promoting wholesome relationships and enhancing sexual health. To help men traverse their emotional landscapes and strengthen their close relationships, we will examine practical communication skills and delve into an understanding of emotions in this chapter.

Understanding Your Emotion

The cornerstone of emotional intelligence is emotional awareness. It entails acknowledging and comprehending one's emotions, which is necessary for effective emotion management. Social standards prohibit men from expressing their emotions freely, which frequently results in emotional repression. As a result, personal well-being and emotional experiences may become disconnected.

Self-reflection is the first step towards identifying your feelings. Spend time recognising your feelings in different contexts, especially when confronted with intimacy and self-worth issues. Journaling might be a valuable tool for this. After critical encounters, especially those involving sexual health, write down your feelings and thoughts. This exercise aids in both pattern recognition and emotional processing.

It's also important to comprehend how emotions and bodily reactions are related. For example, anxiety may result in physiological responses that impair sexual performance, such as tense muscles and elevated heart rate. Understanding these reactions will help you better control your anxiousness and have a more composed attitude during private moments.

The Role of Emotional Awareness in Relationships and Sexual Health

Improving relationships is greatly aided by emotional intelligence. You can react to your partner's sentiments more sympathetically if you know your emotions. Intimacy is based on a deeper emotional connection, which this knowledge fosters. For instance, by admitting that you are nervous before performing, you can talk to your spouse about it instead of having it fester inside of you. You may foster an atmosphere of understanding and support by letting your partner in on your emotional state. This can reduce stress and foster trust, turning intimacy from a solitary endeavour into a cooperative experience.

Additionally, you can identify your partner's emotional signs by cultivating emotional awareness. Being sensitive to their emotions can improve closeness and bonding, simplifying overcoming obstacles. This shared knowledge can result in more robust bonds and more satisfying sex.

7 Effective Communication Techniques for Discussing Fears and Desires with Your Partner

Healthy relationships are built on effective communication. It takes openness and vulnerability to talk about desires and worries, especially concerning intimacy.

Here are some strategies to help lead these crucial discussions:

1. Select the Appropriate Time and
   Location:

When discussing delicate subjects, timing is crucial. Choose a quiet, cosy location where both parties are relaxed. Avoid starting these discussions during private times, as this may put more strain on the relationship.

2. Employ "I" phrases:

To communicate your feelings without assigning blame, frame them in "I" phrases. Rather than blaming your spouse for your destructive emotions, consider saying something like, "I feel anxious about our intimacy," rather than, "You make me feel inadequate."

3. Engage in Active Listening:

Speaking and listening are both necessary for effective communication. By paying close attention, you can demonstrate to your partner that you respect their sentiments. You can show interest by nodding, keeping eye contact, and summarising their points. Saying, "I hear you feel anxious too, and I want us to work through this together" is one example.

4. Be Open and Vulnerable:
It takes bravery to express wishes and worries. Even if your feelings make you uncomfortable, be honest about them. Being vulnerable can foster a closer emotional bond and inspire your spouse to express their emotions.

5. Establish Clear Intentions:
Clearly state your intentions before bringing up delicate subjects. To help frame the conversation positively, you could say something like, "I want to share my feelings about our intimacy because I care about our relationship and want us to grow together."

6. Remain composed and patient:
Talking about intimacy might cause intense feelings. Be patient with both your partner and yourself as you approach these discussions composedly. If emotions run high, consider pausing and returning to the discussion later.

7. Review the Discussion:
Developing emotional closeness is a continuous process. After talking about desires and worries, keep checking in with one another. Frequent discussions about emotional health can create a nurturing

atmosphere and make both spouses feel heard.

How to Handle Disagreement with Love

Relationships will inevitably have conflicts, but how you handle them can significantly impact your mental well-being. Try to treat disagreements with compassion and understanding when they occur. Regardless of your differences, respect one another's emotions. You can show that you respect your partner's feelings by stating, "I understand that you feel hurt by what I said, and I'm sorry for that."

Managing your responses in disagreement is another aspect of emotional intelligence. You can exercise self-regulation by stepping back to evaluate your emotions before reacting. It's acceptable to stop the conversation and return to it when you're both more composed if you're feeling overstimulated.

The Importance of Consulting an Expert

Expert assistance can be beneficial if managing emotions and communicating can be difficult. Individual counselling or couples therapy offers a secure setting for examining emotions and improving communication abilities. A qualified therapist can provide techniques, tools, and insights specific to your requirements. Additionally, counselling can offer a safe space for talking about delicate subjects.

Both spouses can express themselves more freely when a third party is present, which can lessen the emotional burden. Therapists can also help you find better routines by identifying underlying problems causing emotional difficulties. In conclusion, Developing emotional intelligence is a life-changing process that improves relationship health and personal well-being.

By developing emotional awareness, men can better comprehend their emotions and react to their spouses. Good communication skills enable people to freely express their desires and worries, strengthening bonds and improving sexual health. As you proceed, remember that developing emotional intelligence is a lifelong process rather than a final goal. By investing in this crucial area of your life, you not only raise your quality of life overall but also improve your intimate connections, opening the door to a more self-assured and satisfying future.

Chapter 5

The Role of Relationships in All These

Our experiences are greatly influenced by our relationships, especially when it comes to close bonds and private struggles like impotence. A solid partnership can boost resilience and confidence by offering understanding, support, and encouragement. In this chapter, we'll look at how to create a solid connection that fosters self-assurance and techniques for dealing with intimacy issues so that you can stay close even when things go tough.

Supporting Each Other: Building a solid partnership that fosters confidence:
The Value of Supporting One Another When both parties feel appreciated and understood, a relationship flourishes. Being able to rely on one another might be crucial

when dealing with issues like impotence. Establishing a space where both partners can share their weaknesses without worrying about criticism is essential. This transparency improves the emotional connection and builds trust.

1. Establishing a Safe Space:

Provide a secure and accepting setting for conversations around intimacy and sexual health. Since vulnerability is greeted with empathy and compassion, encourage one another to express their thoughts and feelings honestly. Because of this safety net, neither partner feels embarrassed or exposed when expressing their wishes, fears, or worries.

2. Frequent Check-Ins:

Arrange for frequent check-ins to talk about your mental health and connection. These discussions can offer chances to gauge each partner's emotional state and deal with any underlying problems before they become more serious. Use these opportunities to acknowledge accomplishments, show appreciation, and voice any worries that may have come up.

3. Acknowledging Success:

Building confidence requires partners to recognise each other's efforts within and beyond the bedroom. Honour minor successes, such as advancements in communication or anxiety management. In addition to rewarding good behaviour, this acknowledgement deepens the emotional bond.

4. Promoting Development:

Support one another in pursuing hobbies and objectives outside of the partnership. Encouraging your partner's independence and self-worth through their endeavours may result in a healthier dynamic. When both spouses are happy in their personal lives, they can contribute great energy to the partnership.

5. Active Listening Techniques:

Listening is an effective way to provide help. Give your partner your undivided attention when they express their emotions as an example of active listening. To ensure you understand and affirm their feelings, repeat what you have heard. This gives them more confidence to share and shows that you respect their viewpoint.

Developing Transparency to Foster Trust:

Transparency is essential for developing trust in a relationship. Talk candidly about your impotence issues and the emotional toll they take on you. Your spouse will better comprehend your experiences and have the chance to provide support if you are honest with them.

1. Talking About Concerns:

Have an honest conversation about intimacy-related issues. Talk about any worries you may have, whether they relate to your performance, your perception of yourself, or the effect on your relationship. Having these conversations helps you align your expectations and goals while fostering intimacy.

2. Sharing Progress:

Keep your spouse informed of your progress while you work on personal growth through mindfulness exercises, lifestyle modifications, or therapy. This openness keeps them informed and supports your active collaboration to address the issues.

3. Establishing Common Objectives:

Establish shared objectives for closeness and sexual well-being. This may involve trying new things together, like attending intimacy seminars or just committing to regularly check in on each other's emotional well-being. Collaborating to achieve common objectives fortifies the relationship and promotes solidarity.

Strategies for Maintaining Closeness During Difficult Times:

In any relationship, intimacy problems can occur, especially when one partner is coping with personal issues or during stressful periods. Maintaining intimacy and connection while navigating these obstacles calls for a proactive strategy.

1. Redefining closeness:

It's critical to reinterpret what closeness in a relationship entails when dealing with impotence. Emotional and mental relationships are just as significant as physical intimacy. Investigate novel forms of intimacy that are not limited to sexual performance. This can entail holding hands, cuddling, or having in-depth discussions.

2. Open Communication Regarding Intimacy:

Talk about how impotence impacts both spouses' perspectives on intimacy. Promote candid discussion of needs, wants, and anxieties. It is essential to approach this discussion with empathy and understanding, stressing that even in cases when sexual performance is questioned, the emotional bond endures.

3. Investigating Other Intimacy Forms:

Take part in activities that foster intimacy without the strain of sexual performance. Try sharing a bath, getting a sensual massage, or perhaps dancing. Without anticipating sexual activity, these encounters might strengthen emotional closeness and facilitate a physical reunion between partners.

4. Practice Understanding and Patience:

It's important to be patient with one another when things get tough. Recognize that both partners might experience anxiety and vulnerability. Establish a setting that encourages a healthy emotional release by making it acceptable to vent frustration or unhappiness.

5. Seek Professional Guidance Together:

Take into account workshops centered on intimacy and sexual health or couples therapy. A qualified therapist may offer direction, lead conversations, and present fresh approaches to intimacy issues. Collaborating in a nurturing setting can strengthen your bonds and promote development.

6. Emphasis on Emotional Closeness:

During difficult circumstances, make a deliberate effort to keep your emotions close. Take part in bonding activities like date nights, mutual interests, or just spending time together without interruptions. Re-establishing an emotional connection helps lessen the strain caused by physical difficulties.

7. Set Boundaries:

Set limits for chats regarding impotence if they become too much to handle. Limiting conversations to specific hours or taking breaks is acceptable. This can help both spouses enjoy times when their relationship is normal and avoid feeling overtaken by the problem.

8. Honour Each Other's Strengths:

In trying times, remember each partner's positive contributions to the partnership. Acknowledge and appreciate each other's strengths in and out of the bedroom. Mutual support is promoted, and the emotional connection is strengthened when you acknowledge and value your partner's special traits. In conclusion, it is impossible to overestimate the importance of relationships in overcoming obstacles like impotence. Couples can build a solid partnership that boosts resilience and confidence by encouraging open communication, understanding, and mutual support.

Patience, empathy, and a dedication to redefining connection in meaningful ways are necessary for navigating intimate problems. Even in the face of difficulties, you may strengthen your emotional connection by being vulnerable with one another and keeping the channels of communication open.

Chapter 6

Utilizing Professional Help and Resources

Seeking expert assistance can be a crucial step towards empowerment and healing when dealing with issues connected to impotence and confidence. Relationship dynamics and personal well-being can be significantly impacted by knowing when to seek help and investigating the various available therapies and treatments. This chapter will offer guidance on identifying when professional help is required and investigating traditional and alternative therapies.

Knowing When to Speak with Therapists or Medical Professionals

Identifying the Symptoms Although getting help can occasionally be difficult, it's crucial to recognize the warning signs that point to the need for professional assistance. Here are a few important indicators:

1. Persistent Problems:

If impotence persists for over a few weeks, it's best to speak with a healthcare professional. While sporadic challenges may be common, ongoing problems could indicate underlying medical conditions that need to be treated.

2. Emotional discomfort:

It's critical to get help if you discover that impotence is causing you to experience severe emotional discomfort, such as anxiety, melancholy, or feelings of inadequacy. Sexual health is influenced by mental health, and healing can be aided by treating emotional difficulties.

3. Effect on Relationships:

Getting aid is critical when impotence starts to stress a relationship. A therapist or counsellor can offer techniques to overcome these obstacles and strengthen your relationship if intimacy or communication declines.

4. Lifestyle variables:

Suppose you're having trouble with lifestyle variables that lead to impotence, such as eating poorly, not exercising, or abusing drugs. In that case, professional advice can help you make healthy changes and enhance your general well-being.

5. Health Conditions:

It's important to speak with a healthcare professional if you currently have any health issues that could impact your ability to have sex, such as diabetes, high blood pressure, or heart disease. They can evaluate the effects of these diseases on your sexual health and provide suitable treatments.

6. Worried About Drug Side Effects:

Don't be afraid to talk to your doctor if you're taking any medications that you think might be influencing your sexual health. They can assist in deciding whether changes or substitutes are required.

How to Know the Right Medical Professional

Knowing what kind of healthcare professional to consult is crucial when getting help. Here are a few choices:

1. Primary Healthcare Physicians:

Your primary care physician may be your initial point of contact. They can perform preliminary examinations, rule out underlying medical conditions, and, if required, send you to specialists.

2. Urologists:

These experts can offer comprehensive assessments of impotence and concentrate on male reproductive health. They can identify particular ailments and provide personalised treatment alternatives.

3. Mental Health Professionals:

Counsellors, psychologists, and sex therapists can assist in addressing the psychological and emotional components of impotence. They can offer a secure environment for discussing emotions, anxieties, and interpersonal dynamics.

4. Endocrinologists:

If hormonal abnormalities are a contributing factor to impotence, an endocrinologist can measure hormone levels and recommend suitable treatment choices.

5. Sexual Health Clinics:

These speciality clinics concentrate on sexual health and may provide a variety of services, such as support groups, medical evaluations, and counselling.

Exploring Holistic Approaches and Medical Options.

Alternative remedies can be used with traditional medical treatments to cure impotence. You can make well-informed decisions that best meet your needs if you know these options. Holistic Methods

1. Meditation and mindfulness:
These techniques can help lower stress and anxiety, two factors that frequently lead to impotence. Deep breathing, progressive muscle relaxation, and guided visualisation are among the techniques that can increase sexual performance and emotional well-being. Including mindfulness in everyday activities can promote serenity and presence, improving sexual health in general.

2. Yoga and Exercise:
Regular exercise, especially yoga, can increase body awareness, decrease stress, and improve flexibility. By focusing on the pelvic floor muscles, several yoga poses enhance sexual function and increase blood

flow to the vaginal area. Furthermore, yoga's mindfulness component promotes self-acceptance, which can increase self-esteem.

3. Nutritional Therapy:
Seeking advice from a dietician or nutritionist can result in customised meal regimens that enhance sexual function and general health. Foods high in vitamins, healthy fats, and antioxidants can support sexual health. Eating a balanced diet improves energy levels, hormone balance, and circulation.

4. Acupuncture:
Thin needles are inserted into specific body locations during acupuncture, an ancient Chinese medical procedure. Acupuncture may enhance sexual performance by improving blood flow and lowering stress, according to some research. If you're thinking about getting acupuncture, look for a licensed professional who has treated sexual health concerns before.

5. Herbal Supplements:
Traditionally, ginseng, ginkgo biloba, and maca root have been used as herbal medicines to improve sexual health. Before beginning any supplements, it's important

to speak with a healthcare professional because they may not be appropriate for everyone and can mix with prescriptions.

Medical Treatment Options

1. Medication:
By increasing blood flow to the penis, several prescription drugs can effectively treat impotence. Among them are PDE5 (phosphodiesterase type 5) inhibitors, which include Levitra, Cialis, and Viagra. To determine if these drugs are right for you and discuss any possible side effects, speak with your healthcare professional.

2. Hormone Therapy:
Hormone replacement therapy, or HRT, may be a possibility if impotence is found to be caused by hormonal abnormalities. In order to increase sexual function and restore equilibrium, this treatment entails taking supplements of testosterone or other hormones. To guarantee safety and effectiveness, a healthcare provider must do routine monitoring.

3. Vacuum Erection Devices (VED):
These devices increase blood flow and produce an erection by creating a vacuum around the penis. Since they are non-

invasive, VEDs can be combined with other therapies.

4. Penile Injections:
Penile injections may be a valuable treatment for impotence in particular men. By boosting blood flow, these drugs, which are injected directly into the penis, cause an erection. When oral medications are contraindicated or ineffective, this approach is usually taken into consideration.

5. Surgical Options:
Surgical procedures could be considered when all other therapies have failed. Impotence can be permanently resolved with procedures like vascular surgery or penile implants. Speaking with a urologist can help you determine if surgery is the right course of action for you.

People can take proactive measures towards recovery by recognising the warning indicators that point to the need for help. Speaking with medical professionals, such as physicians, therapists, and experts, ensures a thorough approach to treating the psychological and physical components of impotence.
Investigating alternative remedies might also offer supplemental assistance in

addition to traditional treatments. Herbal medicines, yoga, nutritional therapy, and mindfulness are examples of holistic practices that help improve sexual health and general well-being.

Medical solutions such as drugs and surgery should also be considered depending on each person's demands and situation. By utilizing the resources and expert advice available, men can deal with the challenges of impotence more resiliently and confidently.

Chapter 7

Rebuilding Your Confidence Back

A key component of conquering obstacles like impotence and improving general wellbeing is regaining confidence. Every element of life is impacted by confidence, which affects self-perception, career pursuits, and interpersonal interactions. This chapter will explore self-improvement strategies, emphasizing goal-setting and acknowledging minor victories. Furthermore, we will examine how pursuing interests and hobbies can empower people by promoting self-worth and self-esteem. Self-Improvement Strategies:

Setting Personal Goals and Celebrating Small Wins.

Establishing personal objectives gives one a sense of purpose and direction and is a potent approach to drive energy towards positive behaviours. By providing a path for personal development, goals help people concentrate on their objectives.

1. SMART Goals Framework:

When setting SMART goals, take into account the SMART criteria—specific, Measurable, Achievable, Relevant, and Time-bound. For example, a SMART goal would be, "I will exercise for 30 minutes, three times a week for the next month," rather than "I want to be healthier." This level of detail makes it simpler to monitor progress and keep motivated.

2. Divide Up Bigger objectives:

Having significant objectives can be intimidating, particularly if you're struggling with confidence. Divide these objectives into more doable, smaller steps. Your minor goals could be going to a workshop, speaking with a healthcare professional, or adding particular activities to your regimen if your main objective is to enhance your sexual health.

Every little step taken makes you feel like you've accomplished something.

3. Put Your Goals in Writing:

Setting goals in writing shows your dedication to them and reminds you of your objectives. Consider establishing a journal in which you can record your objectives, monitor your development, and consider your path. Additionally, this practice might give you a visual record of your progress over time.

4. Set Deadlines:

Giving your goals due dates instils a sense of responsibility and urgency. Whether the objective is long-term (to be accomplished in a year) or short-term (to be performed in a month), having a deadline promotes steady effort. Ensure you're on track by reviewing your work regularly and modifying your timetables. Honouring Minor Victories Rebuilding confidence requires recognizing and applauding minor accomplishments. Every advancement, no matter how small, merits praise. Celebrating successes encourages continuous improvement and reinforces excellent behaviour.

Here are a few successful celebration ideas:

1. Engage in Self-Recognition:

Give your accomplishments, no matter how minor, some thought. Saying anything as essential as "I'm proud of myself for sticking to my exercise routine this week" might help people regain their self-esteem since self-acknowledgment fosters a constructive internal conversation.

2. Share Your Successes with Others:

Sharing your successes with loved ones, friends, or a supportive community can increase the positive emotions associated with accomplishments. Consider talking to someone familiar with your trip about your objectives and significant events. Their support and affirmation can help you feel more confident.

3. Reward Yourself:

Create a system of incentives for reaching significant goals. This could involve taking a day off to unwind and rejuvenate, enjoying a favourite meal, or reading a new book. Anticipating a reward might give a sense of accomplishment and extra motivation.

4. Make a Visual Representation:

To illustrate your objectives and accomplishments, think about making a vision board or a visual progress chart. Add a milestone to your chart each time you achieve it. This physical depiction promotes a sense of accomplishment by continually reminding you of your progress.

5. Evaluate Your Progress:

Make time regularly to consider your progress. Examine your original objectives and contrast them with your present successes. This reflection not only demonstrates your development but also reaffirms that despite obstacles, advancement is achievable.

Engaging in Activities That Foster Self-Esteem

Building activities: Pursuing interests and hobbies is critical to restoring confidence and boosting self-esteem. These pursuits allow people to express themselves, be creative, and interact with others, all of which support a more positive self-image.

Here's how to use interests to empower yourself:

1. Find New Interests:

Trying out new pastimes can be a fun way to learn about yourself. Trying something new can spark passion and enthusiasm, whether painting, cooking, trekking, or learning to play an instrument. Enjoy the chance to try new things and venture outside your comfort zone.

2. Emphasis on Skill Development:

Learning and skill development are frequently a part of engaging in a hobby. This method cultivates a sense of accomplishment in addition to improving competence. You'll probably feel more confident as your abilities advance. For instance, solving a difficult problem or perfecting a new cuisine can give you a sense of achievement.

3. Social Links:

Hobbies frequently offer chances for social contact, which is advantageous for boosting self-esteem. Join groups related to your interests, such as clubs or classes. Rebuilding confidence requires support and a sense of belonging, which can be found by connecting with people with similar interests.

4. Mindfulness and Flow:

Hobbies can help people achieve a level of mindfulness in which they are totally absorbed in the task at hand. While in this "flow" condition, you can momentarily put your anxieties and insecurities aside, which can be helpful. These periods of immersion, whether painting, gardening, or participating in sports, can improve your mood and sense of self.

5. Volunteering & Community Involvement:

Consider setting aside time for volunteer work or community initiatives related to your hobbies. Assisting others cultivates thankfulness and fulfilment, giving one a sense of purpose. Contributing to something greater than yourself can greatly boost one's sense of connection and self-worth.

6. Establish Hobbies-Related Goals:

Similar to personal objectives, hobbies-related goals can increase your sense of achievement. These objectives can offer inspiration and guidance, whether deciding to practice an instrument for several hours each week or striving to finish a particular number of paintings.

7. Think About Pleasure:

Regularly pause to consider the happiness that your pastimes provide you. Consider keeping a hobby-related notebook in which you record your experiences, insights, and happy moments. This reflection further supports the beneficial effects of your interests on your well-being.

8. Include Hobbies in Daily Life:

Try your best to include hobbies in your everyday schedule. Prioritizing these hobbies shows a dedication to self-care and personal development, whether painting after work or running in the morning. In conclusion, regaining confidence is a life-changing process that requires commitment and effort. Implementing self-improvement strategies, such as establishing personal objectives and acknowledging minor victories, can establish a positive feedback loop that boosts self-esteem.

Additionally, pursuing interests and hobbies offers a means of self-expression, social interaction, and skill development—all of which support personal empowerment. Adopting this diverse strategy for boosting self-esteem promotes resilience and a revitalized feeling of self-worth.

Every little step you take, whether accomplishing a goal or enjoying a hobby, adds to the larger fabric of your development. In the end, you can develop a deep sense of confidence that enables you to meet life's obstacles with grace and courage by investing in yourself and prioritising pursuits that bring you joy.

Chapter 8

Real Stories of Men Who Suffered Impotence and How They Overcame It

Feelings of stigma and loneliness can be lessened by realizing that impotence is a common struggle. This chapter will examine true accounts of men who have faced impotence head-on and come out on the other side with a newfound sense of self-assurance. Through case studies and testimonies, we'll discover the tactics they employed and the lessons they found during their transformational journeys. Testimonials and Case Studies Case Study

Case Study 1: Mark

Mark, a 42-year-old marketing professional, became impotent. He was under a lot of pressure to excel both personally and professionally. His self-esteem plummeted, which set off a vicious cycle of anxiety that made his condition worse.

- Open Communication and Therapy:

Mark sought assistance from a sexual health specialist therapist. He discovered how to deal with the underlying worry that was causing his impotence through treatment. To promote understanding and support in their relationship, he also confided in his girlfriend about his difficulties.

- Mindfulness Practices:

Mark integrated mindfulness practices into his daily routine to help him deal with stress. He engaged in deep breathing techniques and meditation, which enhanced his general well-being and assisted him in managing his anxiety.

- Physical Fitness:

Mark committed to consistent exercise. He began running three times a week, which improved his confidence and happiness, as well as his physical condition.

Knowledge Acquired:

- Vulnerability Breeds Strength:

Mark found that talking to his partner about his difficulties improved their connection and helped him feel less alone.

- Mind-Body Connection:

He discovered that conquering impotence required concurrent attention to both physical and mental well-being.

- Support Systems Are Important:

Professional advice and a supportive spouse can have a big impact on the recovery process.

Case Study 2: James

James struggled with impotence at the age of 35 following a devastating split. He was ashamed and felt unworthy, which made his problem worse. He didn't start to regain his confidence until he embarked on a path of self-acceptance.

Techniques Used:

- Journaling and Self-Reflection:

James started keeping a journal to examine his emotions of inadequacy. He was able to express his feelings and realize that his sexual performance had nothing to do with his value as a person, thanks to this practice.

- Taking Part in Hobbies:

James found a way to express himself by using old pastimes like painting and guitar playing. These activities increased his self-esteem, and he was able to rediscover his passions.

- Support Groups:

James discovered he was not alone when he joined a support group for males going through comparable struggles. His experiences helped him build understanding and a sense of community.

Knowledge Acquired:

Redefining Self-Worth: James discovered that his worth goes much beyond having sex. A key component of his path to confidence was accepting himself.

The Value of Expression:

James could analyse his feelings and rediscover happiness outside of romantic relationships by participating in creative endeavours.

- Community Support:

Locating a community of similar values offered a secure environment for opening up and recovering.

Case Study 3: David

David's Journey Towards Holistic Recovery After being diagnosed with diabetes, 50-year-old businessman David began to experience impotence. At first, he felt helpless when confronted with a chronic illness. But he decided to take charge of his health by adopting a comprehensive strategy.

Techniques Used:

- Nutritional Adjustments:

To create a balanced diet that met his health requirements, David sought advice from a nutritionist. He emphasised eating more fruits and vegetables, cutting back on sugar, and focusing on complete meals.

- Exercise and Weight Management:

To assist control his diabetes and enhance his general health, he developed a regular exercise regimen that included aerobic and strength training activities. 3. Alternative Therapies: David investigated mindfulness exercises and acupuncture, which he found to be beneficial for stress management and enhancing his sexual well-being.

Knowledge Acquired

- Proactive Health Management:

David came to understand that changing his lifestyle to take control of his health had a big impact on his wellbeing and self-esteem. Integration of Approaches: He found that integrating holistic therapies with traditional medical guidance helped him heal. Resilience: David learnt resilience and the value of adjusting to life's obstacles by confronting chronic disease head-on.

Case Study 4: Alan

Alan's Narrative of Rebuilding His Relationship After a challenging period in his relationship, Alan experienced impotence at the age of 29. Their connection was further harmed by a vicious cycle of performance anxiety brought on by the emotional strain. Alan was aware that he had to deal with the problem for the sake of his relationship as well as himself.

Techniques Used:

1. Couples Therapy: In order to address the effects of impotence on their relationship and to have a forum to freely express their

thoughts, Alan and his partner sought couples' therapy.

- Intimate Adjustment

They discovered how to reinterpret intimacy in a way that goes beyond sexual performance. Their emotional connection grew stronger as they started experimenting with non-sexual forms of communication, like holding hands and snuggling.

- Communication and Education

By learning about impotence and its causes, they were able to allay anxieties and misconceptions. They made sure they could talk about their wants and worries without feeling embarrassed by practicing open communication.

Knowledge Acquired

The Power of Open Communication: Alan learnt that communication is essential to a relationship's intimacy and connection. Emotional Connection Is Vital: In difficult times, re-establishing emotional intimacy is frequently more crucial than re-establishing physical closeness.

Professional Advice:

Consulting a therapist can give you the skills and techniques you need to handle challenging conversations and strengthen your bond.

In conclusion Mark, James, David, and Alan's travels show the various routes people can follow to get over impotence and regain their confidence. Every narrative emphasises how critical it is to treat this challenge's emotional as well as physical aspects.

Important Takeaways

- Vulnerability and Support:

Talking about difficulties with dependable people or in support groups promotes comprehension and recovery.

- Holistic Approaches

A complete plan for conquering impotence can be developed by combining alternative, emotional, and physical therapy.

- Redefining Self-Worth

People can rediscover their identities outside of sexual performance by focusing on self-acceptance and taking up hobbies.

- Communication is Key

Honest discussions about wishes and worries can improve bonding and lessen partnership anxiety. These true tales and methods are potent reminders that conquering impotence is a process of self-awareness, grit, and personal development rather than only treating a medical condition.

The fundamental ideas of support, communication, and self-acceptance are ubiquitous in regaining intimacy and confidence, even though each person's path may be unique.

Chapter 9

The Future of Empowerment

Our perceptions of confidence, masculinity, and the intricacies of sexual health change along with society. The path to empowerment is not only individual but also communal, cultivating a culture that values development and accepts vulnerability. This chapter will examine changing ideas about masculinity and the value of establishing a support community for further empowerment.

Changing Views of Masculinity

Redefining the Concept of an Empowered Man Stoicism, domination, and the repression of vulnerability have historically been linked to masculinity. Nonetheless, current debates are moving toward a more complex interpretation of what it means to be an empowered guy.

This reinterpretation promotes authenticity, emotional intelligence, and a broader notion of strength.

1. Accepting Vulnerabilities:

Traditional masculinity frequently views vulnerability as a weakness. Nevertheless, it is among the best qualities a man can have. Men can develop stronger bonds with others and with themselves by accepting vulnerability. The following are some strategies for incorporating vulnerability into the contemporary idea of masculinity:

- Genuine Self-Expression

Empowered men are learning to communicate their feelings without worrying about criticism. By discussing their challenges, anxieties, and insecurities, they can develop a deeper understanding of themselves and strengthen their relationships with others.

- Seeking Assistance:

A key component of contemporary masculinity is admitting when one needs assistance. Men who feel empowered are more willing to ask for help in counselling, support groups, or even casual chats with friends.

- Redefining Success:

External accomplishments, such as wealth, physical prowess, or career standing, are frequently linked to success. The empowered man understands that self-acceptance, wholesome relationships, and emotional health are all necessary for real success.

2. Taking Stereotypes to Task The process of redefining masculinity entails aggressively opposing social norms and stereotypes that prescribe appropriate behaviour for men. This includes:

- Destroying Toxic Masculinity

Toxic masculinity encourages negative attitudes and actions, like emotional repression and aggressiveness. Men can take action to promote healthy behavioural patterns by candidly discussing these ideas and their implications.

Expanding Roles:

The empowered modern man knows that traditional roles are changing, whether related to work, relationships, or parenthood. More and more men are taking up nurturing, housework, and caring duties, upending long-held beliefs and improving family relationships.

- Promoting Inclusivity

Embracing diversity and inclusivity is another aspect of redefining masculinity. Because they understand that masculinity is a continuum with many different expressions rather than a single notion, empowered men appreciate the value of recognising all identities and experiences.

3. Emotional Intelligence

How to Develop Emotional Intelligence A key component of empowered masculinity is emotional intelligence (EQ). It includes the capacity to identify, comprehend, and control one's emotions and those of others. Men can cultivate emotional intelligence in the following ways:

- Self-Reflection

Routinely considering one's feelings and responses can improve self-awareness. Journaling, meditation, and talking with close friends can help.

- Empathy

Comprehending and feeling others' emotions can cultivate deeper ties. Empowered men actively listen to and validate the feelings of others to foster an atmosphere of trust and support.

- Effective Communication

Good relationships depend on expressing ideas and emotions clearly and concisely. Empowered men practice being upfront about their needs and wants, which improves relationships and lessens miscommunication.

Establishing a Support Community

A supportive community greatly aids the development of empowerment. It gives men a safe place to talk about their struggles, victories, and experiences, eventually fostering individual growth and group healing.

- Creating Support Communities

There might be a sense of solidarity in support groups designed especially for guys dealing with problems like impotence, relationship problems, or mental health difficulties. Here are some strategies for creating successful support groups:

- Facilitated talks:

Assign knowledgeable facilitators to lead talks and keep them on-topic and constructive. They can present subjects that promote a more thorough examination of feelings and experiences.

- Frequent Meetings

Establishing a solid support system requires consistency. Establishing frequent meetings, whether in person or virtually, can maintain relationships and encourage continued support.

- Making Use of Technology

To Connect: In the current digital era, technology can establish and maintain supportive groups.

- Online Forums and Groups:

Establishing specific areas on social media sites like Facebook or Reddit might encourage conversations among men dealing with comparable issues. These discussion boards can be secure places to exchange stories and seek guidance.

- Webinars and Workshops:

Organizing online workshops that cover subjects like sexual wellness, emotional health, and masculinity may build community and offer valuable tools. These meetings may include specialists, special guests, or testimonies from guys who have overcome comparable obstacles.

- Apps for help:

For guys looking for help, mental health and wellness apps can provide tools, resources, and coping mechanisms. Features like community forums, meditation activities, and journaling prompts can improve personal development.

- Promoting Peer Mentoring:

A key component of empowerment and personal growth is mentoring. Putting in place a peer mentorship program can help people form deep connections. Connecting Mentors and Mentees:

Assign guys who have overcome obstacles to people with difficulty right now. This connection promotes a feeling of possibility and hope by enabling the exchange of tactics, knowledge, and insights.

Mentor Training:

Offering mentors training can increase their efficacy. Concentrate on their communication, empathy, and active listening abilities to ensure they can provide sincere help.

- Putting Together Community Events

Bringing mentors and mentees together helps strengthen bonds and promote a feeling of community. Workshops, retreats, and casual get-togethers are examples of these events.

- Increasing Advocacy and Awareness

Increasing advocacy and knowledge of men's health issues is another aspect of building a supportive community. Here's how to participate: Educational initiatives: Dispelling myths and educating others can be achieved by starting initiatives that tackle the stigma associated with emotional fragility and impotence. To raise awareness, use workshops, social media, and neighbourhood gatherings.

Participating in Community Service:

Promote group participation in community service initiatives that support mental health and overall well-being. Volunteering together can improve society and deepen relationships.

In conclusion, Redefining masculinity and creating supportive networks are key to the future of empowerment. Empowered men embrace diversity, emotional intelligence, and vulnerability as cultural views change. By questioning conventional wisdom and supporting more positive manifestations of masculinity, men may create stronger bonds and rethink what it means to be strong.

These initiatives are strengthened by the establishment of encouraging communities which offer secure settings for communication, development, and mentoring. Men may create networks that promote resilience and continuous empowerment by starting support groups, using technology, and raising awareness.

It's critical that we carry on these discussions and encourage one another as we progress towards improved mental health, self-acceptance, and true masculinity. By working together, we can establish a world where every man can be himself and form deep connections.

Conclusion

The Path Forward As we conclude this investigation into empowerment, it is critical to acknowledge that the path to self-improvement, self-assurance, and conquering obstacles such as impotence is a continuous one. Empowerment is an ongoing process that calls for dedication, introspection, and fortitude; it is not a destination.

The Path Ahead:

An Ongoing Procedure The road to empowerment is frequently not a straight line, and life is full of ups and downs. The ideas and techniques offered in this book are not just things to cross off a list; they are tools to use in your life as you deal with different obstacles. No matter how good or bad, every event helps you grow. Accepting this journey entails realizing that while setbacks may happen, they do not determine your potential or value.

Remember that every move you take, no matter how tiny, will bring you one step closer to becoming a more powerful version of yourself as you build emotional intelligence, rethink your ideas about masculinity, and interact with encouraging communities. Honour your accomplishments, reflect on your past, and be open to new ideas and development.

Think carefully about the changes you wish to make in your life. Every action you do to improve your well-being counts, whether joining a support group, going to therapy, or having candid discussions about your emotions.

Make connections with others who can relate to your path, exchange experiences, and gain knowledge from one another. By working together, you can create an atmosphere of empowerment where people feel supported and empathetic when they show vulnerability.

Finally, remember that every person's path to empowerment is different. Accept your path, make concrete changes, and don't hesitate to ask for help when needed. As you proceed, take with you the understanding that empowerment is possible and a continuous process.

www.ingramcontent.com/pod-product-compliance
Lightning Source LLC
Chambersburg PA
CBHW050822250726
48653CB00006B/2367